A GUIDE
TO
SLIMMING
AND
HEALTHY
FOOD

DR. MUNEER AL-ALI

(Third Edition)

2024

Third Edition 2024 (B&W)

ISBN-13: 979-8-6290-5976-9

Kindle Direct Publishing - Amazon

Contents

Author

Dr Muneer Al-Ali FRCS (Ed.) is a consultant urological and transplantation surgeon and former professor of urology. He published numerous medical articles in academic journals, and has contributed to, many medical reference books. Al-Ali is also an affiliate scholar at School of Divinity, University of Edinburgh, United Kingdom. He published a few books in both English and Arabic, and contributed to English and Arabic Wikipedia.

Preface

Subjects of this book are based on recent studies conducted by researchers in the fields of medicine, nutrition and public health, from various international universities, institutions and specialised websites. I have vetted the authenticity of the subjects' references.

This book has the advantage of simplifying the scientific jargon and giving a concise summary of the studies, "spot on" information and discusses issues, which urgently require a paradigmatic shift in our understanding of healthy nutrition, life-style and slimming.

Dr Muneer Al-Ali, FRCS

Edinburgh- UK

March 2020

Three Surprisingly Slimming Foods

Memorial Day weekend heralds the official start of bathing suit season -- but it doesn't have to mean the end of delicious meals and snacks! There are tons of yummy foods that will actually help you lose weight, rather than sabotaging your efforts. Here are three stay-slim foods that just might surprise you.

1. Curry

Do you love a great Indian or Thai curry? Good! Because those dishes are prepared with hot chili pepper, which contains a metabolism-reviving ingredient called capsaicin. According to SELF contributing editor Janis Jibrin, a registered dietician, capsaicin offers a "double boost" to your weight-loss efforts.

Research from Aarhus University in Denmark, published in the Journal of Biological Chemistry, shows that capsaicin consumption was associated with an increase in thermogenesis (the process by which cells convert energy into heat), which boosts body temperature and the metabolism. "It encourages your body to burn more calories," Jibrin explains, "and, according to the research, it may also help suppress appetite."

Just make sure to steer clear of creamy curry sauces, because they can defeat the slimming components of the hot chili.

2. Cheese

Jibrin says that although it's calorie-dense (especially full-fat cheeses), studies show that cheese-eaters tend to be thinner! As SELF previously reported, a study in The American Journal of Clinical Nutrition showed that women who ate an ounce of full-fat cheese daily gained fewer pounds over time than their less-cheesy peers. A possible explanation is that whole dairy contains conjugated linoleic acid, which may stoke your metabolism. But, keep in mind -- that's only eating one ounce -- not a lot.

Jibrin points to other studies that show consumers of ALL dairy products are thinner, which, she says, may be because of the calcium. "One theory," she says, "is that when you're deficient in calcium, your appetite increases in the hopes that if you eat more, you'll take in more calcium." Jibrin says low-fat cheeses are your best bet for weight loss. "Stick to about 2-3 ounces daily," she recommends, "and try to keep the rest of your meal low in saturated fat, which cheese is notoriously rich in."

3. Nuts

Although nuts are high in calories and so should be eaten in moderation, the calories in nuts come mainly from their high levels of monounsaturated fats, which are extremely good for health. Eating foods rich in these fats can help reduce bad cholesterol and lower your risk of heart disease and stroke. As well as their heart benefits, nuts are also a great source of protein and are packed with fibre, antioxidants, fatty acids and vitamins and minerals. It is worth noting that peanuts are actually legumes and have different nutritional properties from tree nuts, but there are many other good options to pick from including *Brazil nuts, cashews, walnuts, pecans and pistachios.*

"Let's count the ways," says Jibrin. "First, relative to other foods, nuts are highly satiating, meaning you feel fuller, longer for the calories," she says. Research from the University of Barcelona, published in the American Chemical Society's Journal of Proteome Research, found that eating mixed nuts increases your serotonin levels (one of your "feel-good" neurochemicals), which improves your mood, decreases your appetite and is good for your heart!

And, a study from Purdue University, Indiana, published in the International Journal of Obesity, found that when study participants added about 500 calories' worth of peanuts to their diets, not only did they eat less at subsequent meals, but their metabolisms revved up by 11 per cent. This brings us to Jibrin's second point: "Compared to other foods, nuts tend to increase calorie burn after eating them." She adds, "You don't fully absorb them, so some of the nuts leave your system -- along with their calories."

The 3 Day Tummy Trimming Diet Plan

We women are putting our health at risk with our wobbly tummies. But no more! Follow …

Women have always battled the old waistline, but new findings show we're all creeping over the healthy mark and need to get those tummies in check for the good of our health.

The average waist size for women in the UK is 4.9cm larger than recommended as healthy, the new research has found.

The survey of 54,000 women carried out by Britain's largest healthcare charity Nuffield Health shows that the vast majority of women assessed had a waist size in the 'high health risk' category.

Not only does this not look great in your bikini, but carrying weight around your middle significantly increases the risk of breast cancer, infertility, not to mention heart and liver disease and type (2) diabetes. Cripes!

So, what's the key to a trimmer tummy?

Nutritional Therapist, Alison Stork from Nuffield Health recommends a diet that delivers a full range of important vitamins and minerals, which will help keep you full and regulate fat storage.

Try Alison's three day tummy trimming plan to kick start that waist weight loss:

Day 1

Breakfast

Porridge with a tablespoon of crushed, mixed seeds (pumpkin, linseed, sunflower)

Lunch

Vegetable and Lentil Soup

Dinner

Grilled Salmon with salad and new potatoes

Snacks

Plain yoghurt with fresh fruit

Day 2

Breakfast

Boiled Egg with a slice of wholemeal toast

Lunch

Jacket sweet potato with hummus and mixed salad

Dinner

Stir fry chicken & vegetables with brown rice

Snacks

Fresh Fruit and a small handful of unroasted, unsalted nuts

Day 3

Breakfast

Fresh fruit with plain yoghurt and a dessertspoon of mixed nuts & Seeds

Lunch

Sardines on toasted rye or wholegrain bread with grilled tomato and a sprinkle of herbs & green salad.

Dinner

Lentil Dahl with mixed steamed vegetables

Snacks

Oatcake with cottage cheese

We're on it! Slimmer tummies here we come…

7 Secrets to Getting a Flat Tummy (Without Exercise)

That washboard stomach still eluding you? Try a few !

For women particularly the tummy can be a very difficult place to lose weight. Even if you're hitting the gym and eating right you can still suffer a paunch that just won't shift.

So sometimes, you need to employ some non-exercise based tricks to really see the difference. Try these flat tum hacks for a stomach that would make Cara D jell.

Sleep More

Yes, this is a bonafide tummy-shrinking tip. Of course being asleep means you can't snack (unless you're a sleep walking fridge picker), but also sleep regulates your hormones, especially those caused by stress. By giving your body the chance to deal with stress better you won't be so likely to reach for a high-sugar snack when you're frazzled. And because the cortisol your body reduces when stressed messes with insulin it'll help keep your blood sugar stable - key to a flat stomach.

So if you skipping sleep in favour of the gym you might actually be doing yourself a disservice. Aim for 7-8 hours a night and give your body a break if you need it.

Stand Up Straight

If you want to slim down your stomach, stand up straight. Slight tweaks to your posture can make all the difference. Standing correctly – up tall with your head held high – has an instant slimming effect and encourages you to walk with confidence. By naturally drawing your tummy in, you strengthen your core without realising. And if this focus on your posture has inspired you to take further steps to weight loss success, try Pilates. It's a far cry from intense sessions on the cardio machines, and leaves you feeling spiritually in tune. Stretch your way to a slimmer you.

Drink Milk

To beat a rounded tummy, increase your milk intake, say researchers at the *University of Tennessee.* According to the Nutrition Institute, drinking three glasses of milk a day can work wonders when teamed with a reduced-calorie diet. They believe that the calcium and dairy combo helps speed up the metabolism, leaving more room for fat-burning and smaller tums. Worth a try!

Go Shopping

If you've piled on the pounds over winter, going clothes shopping is probably the last thing on your mind. But pick the right wardrobe, and you can look slimmer in seconds. Don't buy clothes that don't fit. If they're too tight, they'll cling to your figure and highlight every bump, whereas baggy clothes are simply unflattering.

Staple items and style proportion are key to looking slim. If you're sporting skinny jeans, balance them out with an oversized jacket. If your dress resembles a potato sack, belt-up for an instant waistline. And remember – accentuate your best bits. Flattering colours such as black draw the eye to all the right places, along with statement jewellery.

Ladies, high-waisted pencil skirts are perfect for disguising problem areas. They cinch the waist and create an enviable hourglass silhouette. Team with killer heels for a quick confidence boost. And for the fellas, dig out the denim – jeans are always super-flattering.

If you're not much of a fashionista, take a friend you trust to tell you the truth about how you look. Add spices to your food to boost your metabolism.

Spice It Up

Turn the heat up a notch with fat-fighting spices. If you're brave enough, flavour your food with some super-hot cayenne pepper – it's said to shrink fat tissues and supress your appetite, leaving the tummy nice and flat in time for spring. And if that doesn't hit the spot, give cinnamon a try – it's great for the metabolism. By adding it to your meals, you can help reduce blood sugar and cholesterol levels. But don't sweat it; you don't have to go spicy. A clove of garlic can also improve your metabolism and eliminate fat from cells.

Guzzle Some Grapefruit

Celebs including Brook Shields and Kylie Minogue swear by the grapefruit diet, but why? Eating half a grapefruit before every meal is said to boost the metabolism and leave you feeling fuller for longer – ideal for secret eaters. Teamed with a hearty morning brekkie, grapefruit could be your ticket to a manageable calorie-controlled diet. Low in calories and high in nutrients; if you can bare the bitter taste, this superfood is a great addition to the breakfast table.

Laugh It Off

When you're feeling down about the extra weight you've put on over Christmas, just laugh it off. According to research made by the *International Journal of Obesity*, it not only brightens the mood, but it also burns calories. By sticking on your favourite comedy and having a good giggle, you can "increase both your heart rate and calorie expenditure by up to 20 per cent." Think of it as a cardio workout on the inside. A happy you , equals a healthier you – flat tummy included.

Top 5 Foods Help You Sleep

Dairy products

If you're struggling to get a good night's sleep, foods containing tryptophan should be a first port of call. Tryptophan, an essential amino acid, helps to raise serotonin and melatonin levels in the body, both of which can help induce sleep. While turkey is a famously good source of tryptophan, other (perhaps more bedtime-friendly) sources include dairy products such as yoghurt and milk.

On top of their tryptophan levels, dairy snacks are also a great source of calcium, which helps the brain to use tryptophan to create melatonin. Research has also suggested that a deficiency of calcium in the diet can cause disturbed sleep patterns and a lack of deep (REM) sleep.

Oats

While many of us associate oats with breakfast time, they are also the perfect evening snack. Oats are a good natural source of melatonin, which is often taken as a sleep aid due to its ability to help regulate the body's internal clock. They are also another good source of tryptophan, especially when combined with milk.

Furthermore, oats are rich in both calcium and magnesium; two minerals that have been proven to promote good quality sleep. For a warm, soothing snack before bed, try eating a small bowl of porridge to help you drift off, combined with any of the following toppings to help double its effects.

Bananas

If you suffer from muscle spasms or cramps during the night, it may be that you are deficient in the electrolytes magnesium and potassium, both of which help to relax muscles and keep them functioning properly. Fortunately, bananas are excellent source of both minerals, making them a good bedtime snack, particularly after a heavy exercise session.

As well as being rich in these essential minerals, bananas also contain tryptophan, which can help to promote sleep. Researchers from the University of New England in New South Wales have also found that having a banana before bed can help sufferers of sleep apnoea by keeping their throats open and therefore reducing the risk of choking.

Cherries

For those who have trouble sleeping, you may be familiar with over-the-counter melatonin supplements used to treat insomnia. However, while melatonin can help to regulate sleep, it may be unwise to rely on supplements for long-term use. Fortunately, cherries provide a great natural source of melatonin as well as being excellent for overall health.

A research study published in *The Journal of Sleep and Sleep Disorders Research* has indicated that consuming tart cherries before bed helped participants sleep faster and easier, making fresh cherries or cherry juice a great natural sleep aid.

Flax seeds

Flax seeds are great for increasing levels of sleep-regulating substance serotonin in the body due to their high levels of both tryptophan and omega-3 fatty acids. Furthermore, the omega-3 fatty acids they contain have been proven to help reduce the anxiety, depression and stress which are leading causes of insomnia, and have been shown to be effective against the condition sleep apnoea.

Not only that, flax seeds are a good source of magnesium, which is renowned for its ability to reduce stress due to its relaxing effect on the muscles and nervous system. Magnesium has also been shown to help prevent restless leg syndrome and night terrors; both of which can affect sleep.

Top 5 Most Addictive Foods

While we all know about the dangers of alcohol, drugs and cigarettes, did you know that you could become addicted to your favourite food? From withdrawal symptoms to changes in brain chemistry, our snacks have surprising ways of keeping us wanting more. Here is our guide to five of the world's most addictive foods.

Chocolate

Many people claim to be chocoholics, but can you really be addicted to chocolate? The answer is... perhaps. One reason many people feel "addicted" to chocolate is that the food's chemical compounds (including theobromine, phenethylamine, anandamide and tryptophan) actually have pleasure-inducing effects that can mimic the effects of drugs on the brain. Chocolate also contains alkaloids (tetra-hydro-beta-carbolines) which are present in alcohol and have been linked to alcoholism.

However, before you go booking yourself into Chocoholics Anonymous - it is important to note that many researchers have pointed out that the chemicals in chocolate also exist in other foods which most of us do not crave. It has also been suggested that the chemicals in chocolate are not in high enough doses to lead to addiction. Regardless, it is impossible to deny that chocolate is one of the world's most-craved foods - whether this is due to psychological reasons or a physical addiction.

Cheese

From pizzas to cheeseburgers, cheese is a staple of many widely-craved junk foods, but there could be more to our cravings than we think. Various studies have discovered the presence of opiates - including the highly addictive morphine - in the popular dairy product.

While the amounts of morphine in cheese are very small and probably not enough to cause addiction, some researchers have expressed concern about its levels of casein (the main protein in cheese) which produces morphine-like opiate compounds called casomorphins during digestion. On top of this, cheese also contains phenyl ethylamine, a substance with stimulant effects which is thought to give consumers a natural "high", and which is reputed to have addictive qualities.

Sugar

We all know that sugar is bad for our health but, according to numerous studies, it can also be addictive. Studies have suggested that when we eat sugar, chemicals called opioids are released by the brain, which leads to an intense feeling of pleasure. It is this feeling that people may crave in the absence of sugar.

A study by psychologists at Princeton University investigated sugar addiction by studying its effect on rats. They discovered that after rats were fed a diet high in sugar, they experienced symptoms similar to those produced by drug withdrawal when the sugar was withdrawn, including shaking and changes in brain chemistry. The study therefore concluded what other researchers have also suggested; that it is possible to become severely dependent on sugar.

Burgers and other processed meat

Numerous researchers and studies have suggested that fatty, processed junk food such as burgers may actually be addictive. According to Professor David Kessler - an ex-commissioner of the US Food and Drug Administration and author of *The End of Overeating* - the combination of fat, salt and sugar in junk food triggers our "bliss point" and leaves us wanting more.

Scientists at the Scripps Research Institute in Florida backed up this theory with a study which found that the addictive responses in the brains of rats when fed junk food including fatty meats were the same as in those that consume cocaine or heroin. On top of this, meat - like chocolate, cheese and sugar - releases opiate-like substances during digestion which some studies have suggested can leave us craving more.

Coffee

Many feel that they can't start the day without a cup of coffee and people often joke about having a caffeine "addiction", however this may not be far from the truth. Although there has been much debate over the years about whether or not caffeine is genuinely addictive, it is difficult to deny that many of us crave it to the point where we feel we can't function without it.

One reason that people may crave caffeine so much is due to the fairly severe symptoms of caffeine withdrawal that people often face, ranging from fatigue and headaches to irritability and depression. However, it may be that, rather than being physically dependent on caffeine, you are actually addicted to the belief that you can't function without your morning cup of coffee. Whatever the reason , caffeine remains the world's most popular drug and a staple of many daily routines.

Top 10 Detox Foods

10 cleansing foods to get your body back on track

Recently overindulged? Feeling a bit sluggish? Or just not looking your best? It could be that your body is in need of a detox. Fortunately, there are many foods around that can help counteract the effects of a toxic lifestyle. Whether you want to lose weight, feel more energised, improve your complexion or boost your mood, check out these top 10 foods to cleanse your body and boost your health.

1-Lemon

Lemons are a staple of many detox diets, and there is good reason for this. Firstly, lemons are packed with antioxidant vitamin C, which is great for the skin and for fighting disease-forming free-radicals. Furthermore, the citrus fruit has an alkaline effect on the body, meaning that it can help restore the body's pH balance, benefitting the immune system. Try starting your day with hot water and a slice of lemon , to help flush out toxins.

2-Ginger

If too much fatty food or alcohol has caused problems for your digestive system, it may be worthwhile adding some ginger to your diet. Ginger is not only great for reducing feelings of nausea, but it can help improve digestion, beat bloating and reduce gas. In addition to this, ginger is high in antioxidants and is good for boosting the immune system. To give your digestion a helping hand, try sipping on ginger tea or adding some freshly grated ginger to a fruit or vegetable juice.

3-Garlic

Garlic has long been known for its heart benefits; however the pungent food is also good at detoxifying the body. Garlic is not only antiviral, antibacterial and antibiotic, but it contains a chemical called Alicen which promotes the production of white blood cells and helps fight against toxins. Garlic is best eaten raw, so add some crushed garlic to a salad dressing to boost its flavour and your health at the same time.

4-Artichoke

If you have recently been overindulging in fatty foods and alcohol, adding some steamed globe artichoke leaves to your meals is a great way to help get your body back on track. Globe artichokes are packed with antioxidants and fibre and can also help the body digest fatty foods. On top of this, globe artichoke is renowned for its ability to stimulate and improve the functions of the liver - the body's main toxin-fighting tool.

5-Beetroot

For those needing a quick health-boosting shot of nutrients, you can't do much better than beetroot. Packed with magnesium, iron, and vitamin C, the vegetable has recently been hailed as a superfood due to its many reported health benefits. Not only is beetroot great for skin, hair and cholesterol levels, but it can also help support liver detoxification, making it an ultimate detox food. To enjoy its benefits, try adding raw beetroot to salads or sipping on some beetroot juice.

6-Green tea

While it's not technically a food, no detox plan would be complete without regular consumption of essential liquids. Fluids are essential for keeping our organs healthy and helping to flush toxins from the body, and drinking green tea is a great way of boosting your intake. Green tea is not only a good weight-loss drink, but it is extremely high in antioxidants. Research has also suggested that drinking green tea can protect the liver from diseases including fatty liver disease.

7-Cabbage

Many celebs have resorted to the cabbage soup diet to help lose weight and get in shape quickly before a big event, however cabbage is not only good for weight loss - it is also an excellent detoxifying food. Like most cruciferous vegetables (including broccoli and sprouts), cabbage contains a chemical called sulforaphane, which helps the body fight against toxins. Cabbage also supplies the body with glutathione; an antioxidant that helps improve the detoxifying function of the liver.

8-Fresh fruit

Fresh fruits are high in vitamins, minerals, antioxidants and fibre and are also low in calories, making them an important part of a detox diet. If you're after brighter eyes and skin, shinier hair and improved digestion, try boosting your intake of fruit and eating from a wide variety of different kinds. The good news is fruit is easy to add to your diet, so try starting your day with a fresh fruit salad or smoothie and snacking on pieces of fruit throughout the day.

9-Brown rice

If you want to cleanse your system and boost your health, it is a good idea to cut down on processed foods. Instead, try supplementing your diet with healthier whole grains such as brown rice, which is rich in many key detoxifying nutrients including B vitamins, magnesium, manganese and phosphorous. Brown rice is also high in fibre, which is good for cleansing the colon, and rich in selenium, which can help to protect the liver as well as improving the complexion.

10-Watercress

Like most green herbs and vegetables, watercress is an excellent health-booster and detox food. Firstly, watercress leaves are packed with many vital detoxifying nutrients, including several B vitamins, zinc, potassium, vitamin E and vitamin C. Secondly; watercress has natural diuretic properties, which can help to flush toxins out the body. To reap the benefits of this nutritious food, try adding a handful of watercress to salads, soups and sandwiches.

Top 10 Foods That Can Help You Lose Weight

Losing weight is not just about reducing food intake and cutting things out of your diet, there are a few additions that you can make to your daily diet that can indeed help you lose weight. We've found 10 foods, stuffs that incorporated with a healthy eating approach can help you shift those extra pounds and speed up weight loss.

Grapefruit

We've all heard of the grapefruit diet but you don't have to live on a diet of grapefruit alone to lose weight. It's been found that that eating half a grapefruit before each meal or drinking a serving of the juice three times a day can help you drop the pounds. The magic ingredient is the fruit's phytochemicals and their effect of reducing insulin levels which stimulates your body to convert calories into energy rather than storing as flabby fat.

Cinnamon

Cinnamon is a super spice when it comes to boosting your wellbeing as it has many health-giving properties. In terms of weight loss, it's all to do with controlling those post-meal insulin spikes, which is what make you feel hungry. And you don't need to get much of the stuff to get the benefits; studies have shown just a quarter teaspoon of cinnamon a day can lower the blood sugar, cholesterol, and triglyceride levels. To up your cinnamon intake either sprinkle it on to your breakfast cereal, or maybe mix it into your morning latte.

Chilli peppers

Adding a bit of heat to your diet can give you a weight-loss boost. Studies show that having a spicy start to your morning, i.e. eating chillies as a part of your breakfast can make you opt for a smaller lunch. Apparently it's down to capsaicin which is found in chillies and red peppers that has appetite suppressing properties. Granted - chillies aren't the easiest of items to face as your morning meal but how about as a part of a spicy egg-white omelette or stirred into scrambled eggs for a spicy weight loss kick.

Fennel tea

Again fennel tea is a food stuff that boasts a list of health giving benefits; it's packed with good levels of potassium, magnesium and calcium as well as the vitamins B and C. But when it comes to the weight-loss stakes fennel had a double benefit: working both as an appetite suppressant and a metabolism booster which really are both useful if you're trying to lose weight. Fennel tea is widely available in supermarkets so add it to your daily diet to stave off cravings and boost your fuel burn.

Salad

Eating a low-calorie salad before your main meals can help you to lose weight and ensure you get recommended daily intake of veggies. And it's not rocket science as to how it works for weight loss, the key is the sheer volume of a salad, which makes you feel too full to pig out when it comes to your main meal. You need to make sure you don't drown it in a fatty dressing though - a little olive oil and balsamic vinegar makes the perfect healthy accompaniment to a fresh salad.

Green tea

Another powerful brew - green tea really has a multitude of health and wellbeing benefits. And if you are a keen into fitness it makes the perfect pre-workout drink; it's been found to increase endurance by as much as 24%, allowing you to exercise longer and burn more calories. But in terms boosting your weight loss power, a study carried out by the Journal of Nutrition, drinking five cups of green tea per day can help you lose twice as much weight, most of it where you want to lose most , around the middle.

Celery

Celery rates well as a weight-loss food as you can actually end up burning more calories eating it than your body will take on consuming it. But by no means does that make celery low in nutritional value; it's super-packed with fibre (great for digestion) and foliate (the essential nutrient for the care and production of new cells within the body). Get your celery fix by making sure it's featured in your pre-meal salad, as an accompaniment to your lunch or as a healthy snack when you want to satisfy that 'munch' craving.

Lentils

Lentils are great weight-loss food as they have the power to really satisfy your hunger without packing your body with loads of calories and fat - that's often why lentils feature heavily as a meat substitute - they can make you feel like you've had a meaty dish minus the calories and saturated fat that come with eating meat. Again like celery, lentils are full of fibre and foliate so as well as giving you the full feeling, they are great for digestion and healthy cell growth.

Dark chocolate

Granted chocolate is not low in calories nor in fat, but dark chocolate has two major dietary positives that can lead to long term weight loss. First, it's quite difficult to scoff massive quantities of high-quality dark chocolate as compared to the milk stuff. Secondly, dark chocolate is very high in health-promoting antioxidants. In terms of a weapon in your weight-loss armoury you can use dark chocolate as a way to curb any sweet cravings, just a few small squares to quell a full on chocolate pig out is well worth the modest calorie intake.

Quinoa

Pronounced 'Keen-wah', quinoa is known as the 'mother grain' by the ancient Peruvians. Quinoa is good for weight loss as it has the power to keep you feeling fuller for longer due to its high protein content. Also the carbs that are present in the grain are released slowly into the body so you won't get that rush of energy after eating quinoa as you would with other foods like white rice or pasta. You can eat quinoa raw but we reckon it is best when it's cooked in a similar way to rice or couscous.

Top 10 Reasons why you're Not Losing Weight

If you've been adhering to a strict healthy eating and fitness plan for a while but are failing to see the results, it may be time take a look at what is sabotaging your success. From dieting blunders to physical factors, check out the top 10 reasons why you're not losing weight.

You overcompensate for exercise

Many of us are familiar with the temptation to reward our workouts with an edible treat (well, you've just burned off all those calories, right?), however, it may be that by increasing your calorie intake to fuel or reward your sessions you are actually undoing all the hard work of your workout. In fact, as we often overestimate the calories we burn through exercise, you may even be taking in more than you have actually worked off, leading to weight gain rather than loss.

You're not getting enough sleep

You may think that cutting back on sleep to make time for a workout is great for your health and fitness, however not getting enough sleep could actually minimize the benefits of exercise and cause you to gain weight. Not only does sleep deprivation affect exercise performance and endurance, but it slows down your metabolism, increases appetite and makes you more likely to give in to your cravings. Furthermore, lack of sleep can increase stress levels, which can contribute to weight gain.

You're drinking too many sugary drinks

You watch what you eat, cut back on fatty foods and don't snack between meals, but have you considered the amount of calories you may be drinking every day? While we all know the main calorie culprit when it comes to our drinks is alcohol, you should also consider the calories in fruit juice, smoothies, soft drinks and many hot drinks. Every calorie counts towards your daily intake, so don't forget about the liquid ones!

You're eating large portions

If you're eating low fat, healthy meals but are still not losing weight, it may be worth looking at your portion sizes. While you may think that you're only eating three meals a day, with the increasing portion sizes many of us consume you could actually be eating the equivalent of 6 or more standard serving sizes each day. It is worth remembering that although the food you're eating may be healthy, it should still be eaten in moderation, as eating too much of anything will cause you to gain weight.

You're eating too little

While eating too much food can cause you to gain weight, eating too little can also make it surprisingly difficult to shed those pounds. Your body has a natural instinct to protect itself so when it is not given an adequate amount of food it will automatically go into starvation mode, causing the metabolism to slow down and the body to hoard fat and calories. As a result of this it will become much more difficult for you to lose weight.

You're not consistent

Perhaps even worse for your metabolism and waistline than eating too much or too little is flitting regularly between the two extremes. If you constantly take up and abandon faddy diets or go through a process of starving yourself one minute and bingeing the next, you will play havoc with your metabolism and cause your body to store more fat. As eating too little causes the metabolism to slow down, following this period with a binge will cause your body to quickly pile on the pounds.

You don't vary your exercise

If you've fallen into a rut with your exercise routine, you may no longer be getting the most out of your workouts. Not only can doing the same exercise activities over and over cause boredom to set in – which will make you less motivated and more likely to skip your workout – but it will also diminish the intensity and results of your training. As your body becomes more efficient at a certain activity you will no longer need to work as hard at it, meaning that will burn off fewer calories.

You don't need to lose weight

With the growing obesity problem in many parts of the world, it seems as though everybody wants to lose weight. However, although it is a fact that many people do need to shed the pounds, you may not be one of them. Rather than striving for an unrealistic body shape (and remember the lighter you are, the more difficult it will be to shed those pounds), ask yourself – and your doctor –honestly if there are medical reasons you need to lose weight. If not, it may be time to ditch the diet and start giving your self-esteem a workout instead.

Your weight isn't a true reflection of body fat

Many people obsess over their weight as a way of measuring how much body fat they have lost or gained. However, while a set of scales will tell you your weight, it will not tell you how much of that is fat, muscle or water, and therefore is not an accurate representation of fat loss. For instance, gaining muscle through a new fitness routine can slow down weight loss, as can fluid retention. For a more accurate indication of your body fat levels, try tracking changes in your measurements and the fit of your clothes, or get your body fat measured.

You have a medical condition

Many medical conditions such as polycystic ovary syndrome (PCOS), thyroid problems and hormonal imbalances can cause you to gain weight and make it very difficult to lose excess pounds. Also, hidden food allergies or intolerances can make it difficult to lose weight. Furthermore, while your medical condition itself may not cause weight gain, the side effects of certain medications may pile on the pounds, so make sure to speak to your doctor about this if you are struggling to lose weight. Read more on realbuzz.com.

Weight Loss Trends You Should Avoid

Shedding those extra kilos and regaining the perfect physique is a matter of concern for everyone today.

Losing weight is essential, but undergoing this weight loss program the healthy way is extremely crucial. In the frenzy of getting rid of the bulge quickly, one tends to adopt the attractive but unhealthy route. Below are a few weight loss tips that must be avoided:

Diet Pills

Resorting to a number of diet/weight loss pills available in the market is certainly the wrong choice. Watching the so called 'Health Shows' on television, people fall for it and do not question the science behind it which may end up harming the body in the longer run.

Skipping Meals

Skipping meals in the day is definitely the most incorrect way to lose weight. One tends to believe in the notion that avoiding a meal will result in lesser intake of calories, hence loss of weight. Unfortunately such individuals consume more quantity of food in the next meal causing overeating and weight gain instead of loss. So any of you trying to skip your breakfast, lunch or dinner, it's certainly not advisable to do so.

Impatience

Like everything in life, human beings are impatient and expect quick returns and results even with reference to weight loss. It is important to remember that weight loss is a gradual and time-consuming process. Regular exercise, a healthy diet and a patient attitude will eventually show the desired results.

Fasting

A myth that plays around in the minds of people especially the youth today, is that fasting is equal to weight loss. A day or two of fasting cleans and detoxifies the system but continuous lack of food for the body can prove to be a dangerous affair. The body requires a supply of essential vitamins, minerals and fats in order to function. Starvation can invite a number of health problems resulting in the reduction of the immunity levels of the body.

Aggressive exercise regime

Planning and following an aggressive exercise routine is often mistaken with immediate weight loss. What one tends to overlook is the long-term damage done to the body in the tumult of the short-term and immediate results that it produces. A well-planned, disciplined workout regime not only aids systematic weight loss but also boosts energy, improves the overall physical and mental health of the body.

Consuming Diet products and artificial sweetener

Diet snacks, dairy products available in the market certainly facilitate the weight loss process but it is imperative to consume them in moderation as per the diet plan suggested by the expert. Also, artificial sweeteners incorporated in the diet must be consumed in small quantities since anything can excess can be harmful for the body.

Keeping away from these basic pointers will not only help you achieve your weight loss target but also ensure that the process is systematic, not causing any major damages to the body. Stay Fit! Stay Happy!

Top 7 Face-Friendly Foods

Face-friendly food 1: Berries

Berries act as the perfect healthy skin pick 'n' mix as they provide a great combo of antioxidants and vitamins C and E in an easy package. Vitamin C is really face-friendly as it helps produce collagen, the facial framework tissue which keeps your complexion plump and smooth. Blackberries, raspberries, strawberries and blueberries are some of our favourites and easy as to get into your daily diet, but make sure they are eaten fresh and unheated; you'll get the most antioxidants and vitamins that way.

Berries are a great source of skin-friendly nutrients.

Face-friendly food 2: Wholegrains

Wholegrains are a facial super food as they are fantastic for your digestion, and when your body is working to get rid of waste and toxins efficiently it shows on your skin. Go for brown or wholemeal pasta, rice and breads to get your wholegrains as well increase your intake of fibre. These foods not only boost digestive transit, but they are also great sources of iron and another skin-loving nutrient, vitamin B, as well as helping you to feel full and satiated.

Face-friendly food 3: Cucumber

Okay, so you can slice off a couple of rounds and pop them on your eyes too, but the nutritional properties of cucumber make them a skin-friendly food to eat as well. Cucumber has high water content and staying hydrated has to be one of the golden rules when it comes to good nutrition for your skin. Boost your cucumber intake by including them as crudités, in salads and even in drinks - cucumber whizzed up with yogurt, mint and a dash of milk makes a delicious lassie.

Face-friendly food 4: Salmon

Oily fish is super skin-friendly as its rich in the essential lipids (fats) that the skin needs to be healthy. The fatty acid Omega 3 is your friend when it comes to maintaining a healthy and young-looking complexion as it maintains skin elasticity and works to keep cell membranes healthy. Other examples of oily fish include trout, mackerel, tuna, anchovies and sardines.

Face-friendly food 5: Dark leafy greens

Spinach, kale, romaine lettuce, and Swiss chard are all great examples of dark leafy greens that are fantastic for maintaining healthy skin. It's all to do with their super levels of antioxidant, vitamins A, C, E and the mineral iron - which is essential for keeping your blood healthy and your skin bright. If you are not a great lover of greens you can always add them to a smoothie or sneak watercress, rocket or baby spinach into salads and sarnies to ensure you get your fill.

Face-friendly food 6: Beans

It's the existence of isoflaves - potent antioxidants - that make beans a fabulous face-friendly food.

Antioxidants are great because they reduce the free radicals in your body (which cause ageing) and make you look and feel great. And black beans, chickpeas, lentils and soybeans are good choices of beans/legumes to incorporate into your diet.

Face-friendly food 7: Extra virgin olive oil

Integral to the Mediterranean diet, extra virgin olive oil can help nourish your skin from the inside out. High levels of the antioxidant vitamin E and source of the 'good fats' are what make extra virgin olive oil so skin-beneficial. If you don't already, try using it in place of your regular cooking oil and include a drizzle on salads, pasta and pizza.

Jarrah Honey- A Superfood

Source of Jarrah honey

Jarrah honey is a monofloral honey, foraged and collected from the Jarrah flower, a white blossom that blooms in clusters on the Jarrah tree. Jarrah tree (also known as the *Eucalyptus Marginata)* is native to Western Australia in the protected Jarrah wood state forest in the South West of the state. The trees grow up to a towering height of 40 metres. Though the tree itself takes 120 years to grow to full maturity, a Jarrah tree has a relatively long lifespan and can live up to 1,000 years in the wild forests of Western Australia.

Jarrah trees take 2- 3 years to flower, with most of the flowering occurs during springtime. Jarrah tree flower requires sufficient humidity to bloom, which limits its flowering season. Due to its infrequent blooming and crop being affected by extreme weather conditions, such as drought periods, the ability to produce honey is special and deemed a prized product due to its scarcity.

The production process of Jarrah honey is like that of other varieties of honey. The viscous golden liquid is produced when bees forage to extract nectar and pollen from the Jarrah flowers, catalysing the nectar to form a mixture of fructose and glucose which are deposited as honey into the wax cells. With time, and bees hovering over the cells, most of the water in the honey evaporates leaving behind a thick glossy amber liquid with a water content of less than 20%. Its scarcity and impressive health benefits have led to it being dubbed as *"liquid gold"*.

Health benefits of Jarrah honey

For thousands of years, Jarrah honey has been used for its health benefits, which include treating sore throats, wounds, burns etc. as well as being incorporated into people's daily diets for added nutritional value.

1) 1 tablespoon of Jarrah honey on average contains 70 calories, 0.1g of protein, and 17g of

carbohydrates and free of fat. Including honey in a diet, in moderation, has been reported to have cardiovascular benefits, by reducing the harmful LDL *(Low Density Lipoprotein)* levels, triglyceride levels and overall cholesterol levels.[1]

2) One of Jarrah honey's main benefits is its antibacterial properties and general broad-spectrum activity against a wide range of bacterial strains. In addition, some studies reported its effectiveness against antibiotic resistant bacteria strains like MRSA and that it can prevent bacterial growth, with levels as low as12.5% concentration.[2]

Other factors that reinforce its antibacterial properties are:

- Its acidic pH creating a challenging environment for microbes to thrive in.

- Its high sugar and low water content dehydrate bacterial cells. This causes bacterial cell walls to collapse due to osmosis (water moving out of the bacterial cells) resulting in their dehydration and death.

- Bee *Defensin* which is a defense peptide also

believed to contribute to the honey's bacteriostatic properties.

A study suggests that Jarrah honey is effective at limiting bacterial growth. In 8 different pathogenic bacterial strains, Jarrah honey is reported to reduce bacterial growth to 12.5%.[3]

3) As well as being antibacterial, Jarrah honey is also a great source of antioxidants and rich in polyphenols, ascorbic acid (soluble Vitamin C) and flavonoids - all of which are antioxidant sources. The dark amber colour of Jarrah honey indicates the presence of these antioxidant chemicals in any processed batch.[4] Antioxidants work by combating the effects of damaging free radicals which otherwise lead to several harmful effects such as: cell mutations, ageing, cellular damage and many other chronic diseases relating to that of oxidative stress. Environmental stressors contributing to oxidative stress, include exposure to pollutants, smoking, radiation etc.

4) Jarrah honey has been used as an antiseptic for wounds to enhance healing, for more than five thousand years, with its medical-grade derivative being used for wound dressings to treat cuts, burns

and other wounds. Jarrah honey promotes wound healing by creating a moist healing environment. It encouraging tissue repair, as well as inhibiting bacterial growth and prevent infection during the process. A research study from the Department of Agriculture and Food in Western Australia demonstrated Jarrah honey's ability to significantly speed up the healing process of a moderately infected wound in less than one month when being applied twice a day to the affected area [5]. Additionally, research carried out by the University of Auckland, New Zealand reported that honey can be capable of promoting healing faster than conventional dressings do for mild to moderate burns.[6]

5) Jarrah honey also has anti-inflammatory properties, for relieving sore throats of coughs or colds. A study conducted recently showed that the activity levels of enzymes responsible for producing lipids (known as prostaglandins) relating to pain and inflammation decreased as a result of honey.[7] Additionally, honey also decreases the production of *Reactive Oxygen Species (ROS)* which also contribute to inflammation. Studies led by NICE (National Institute of Health and Care Excellence) and PHE (Public Health England) in the UK have

reported the ability of honey to relieve coughs for children over 1 year of age, and is even recommended by the NHS as the first step to consider for treating most acute coughs.[8]

To make a soothing drink for the throat, try mixing 2 tablespoons of lemon juice to a cup of lukewarm water, and adding 1 to 2 teaspoons of Jarrah honey to taste.

Other uses of Jarrah honey

1) Honey helps us detox. Using honey to detox might sound peculiar, but it's really effective! Add honey to water, and add cinnamon, lemon or apple cider vinegar. When you add active, healing honeys to water, make sure you only add it to warm or cool water, to avoiding destroying the delicate enzymes that provide their healing powers.

2) Honey also helps a hangover. When you've overindulged, you might have your go-to remedy of fizzy drinks and carb-loaded pizzas, but next time use honey instead. Honey contains high level of fructose, a type of fruit sugar, than normal table sugar, or glucose. Fructose helps the body break down a by-product of alcohol, called acetaldehyde,

which is the culprit when it comes to hangovers. The quicker we get rid of the acetaldehyde, the quicker we feel fresh again!

Beauty benefits

Unsurprisingly, Jarrah honey also offers benefits in the beauty and cosmetics domain, in addition to its numerous health benefits. Honey is used in a range of beauty and skincare products. It has several desired cosmetic properties, which include cleansers, moisturisers, hair conditioners, shampoos, lip treatments etc. Its anti-inflammatory properties are great for soothing and calming skin, its antibacterial properties utilised for reducing signs of redness and its antioxidising properties used for anti-ageing purposes.

The FDA reports that honey is utilised in over 1,000 registered cosmetic products in the US at a relatively high concentration in those products and up to 22% concentration for face masks.[9]

1) Jarrah honey is packed full of antioxidants with its abundance of flavonoids and polyphenols and is used in cosmetics to visibly reduce signs of ageing. It is used in anti-wrinkle and anti-ageing creams to

achieve more radiant, youthful looking skin. Its antioxidants also help to mitigate the effects of harmful free radicals which could otherwise lead to collagen degradation. It has also been suggested that honey aids with cell regeneration for tissue repair which could aid collagen production and increase skin elasticity.[10]

2) As Jarrah honey has antiseptic properties due to its peroxide content, the honey is incorporated into facial cleansers for visibly reducing the appearance of redness and blotchiness of the skin. Because Jarrah honey contains amino acids, polyphenols, flavonoids, vitamins, and fatty acids, these can contribute to reducing the appearance of uneven skin tone, rosacea and hyperpigmentation. Jarrah honey can be implemented into toners to help soothe and calm the skin, as well as reduce skin irritation due to its anti-inflammatory properties.

3) The high sugar content makes Jarrah honey a great humectant in moisturisers to hydrate the skin, leaving behind more supple skin. Polyphenols in the honey also have water attracting hydrating properties. Improved skin hydration can reduce the appearance of fine lines and wrinkles, as well as allow the skin to appear less dull and leave a natural

dewy glow to your complexion. In addition to its hydrating effect due to its high sugar and polyphenol content, it is also believed that a variety of minerals found in honey (iron, calcium, phosphorus etc.) can contribute to the hydrating property of honey to the skin too.[11]

4) From hair masks for dry hair and split ends, to an exfoliating dry lip treatment and nourishing remedy for brittle nails, honey really ought to be pride of place in our bathroom cabinets as well as our kitchen cupboards. Honey is also wonderful in skin nourishing face masks too, so make sure you add it to your skin care routine.

Beauty tips with Jarrah Honey:

- **A facemask to improve the health and glow of the skin.**

Jarrah honey contains an enzyme which produces hydrogen peroxide. This kills bacteria and therefore, helps to clear spotty skin, and does not cause any inflammation due its anti-inflammatory properties.

The great thing about hydrogen peroxide in Jarrah honey is that it stays active for several days, so not only do existing bacteria die, but more bacteria can't take hold.

Honey is also osmotic. This means that the massive quantities of sugar in it soak up surrounding moisture, killing the bacteria. Again, this means that Jarrah Honey skincare may be ideal if you have spot-prone skin. And by creating a moist healing environment, it helps skin to retain moisture and stay hydrated. This moisturising effect helps with elasticity and the texture of your complexion. The anti-inflammatory effect of Jarrah honey soothes red or inflamed skin and the enzymes.

- **Wound healing and collagen stimulation;** Jarrah Honey induces a marked increase in the regenerative capacity of skin cells, and promotes cell regeneration and collagen production. This remarkable property helps keep skin supple and youthful and can be used as an inti-aging face mask once a week.[12]

- **To treat pimples and acne:** Mix a tablespoon of Jarrah Gold Honey with ½ a teaspoon of cinnamon and apply it to the affected areas – leave on for a few hours before washing off.

- **To treat dry lips:** Apply a thin layer of Jarrah honey to your lips and leave on. Try not to lick it off straight away!

- **To treat enlarged pores and blackheads:** Mix equal parts of lemon juice and Jarrah honey and apply to the affected areas for a few hours and then wash off.
  Lemon juice is a great cleansing compound that works well for skin pores which get enlarged in oily skin, and blackheads, while honey nourishes and balances the skin's pH.

- **For dark spots:** To faint the dark spots and give the skin a healthy glow, mix 1 tablespoonful of Jarrah Gold Honey, 1/4 teaspoonful of Turmeric and a squeeze of lemon, into a paste and apply to the affected areas or use it as a face-mask.

References

1. Anand S, Pang E, Livanos G MN. Characterization of Physico-Chemical Properties and Antioxidant Capacities of Bioactive Honey Produced from Australian

Grown Agastache rugosa and its Correlation with Colour and Poly-Phenol Content. *Molecules.* 2018;23(1):108. doi:10.3390/molecules23010108

2. Al-Waili NS. Natural honey lowers plasma glucose, C-reactive protein, homocysteine, and blood lipids in healthy, diabetic, and hyperlipidemic subjects: comparison with dextrose and sucrose. *J Med Food.* 2004;7:100–107. doi:10.1089/109662004322984789

3. Sushil Anand, Margaret Deighton, George Livanos, Paul D. Morrison, Edwin C. K. Pang NM. Antimicrobial Activity of Agastache Honey and Characterization of Its Bioactive Compounds in Comparison With Important Commercial Honeys. *Front Microbiol.* 2019;10:263. doi:10.3389/fmicb.2019.00263 PMCID: PMC6397887

4. Azhar Sindi, Moses Van Bawi Chawn, Magda Escorcia Hernandez, Kathryn Green, Md Khairul Islam CL& KH. Anti-biofilm effects and characterisation of the hydrogen peroxide activity of a range of Western Australian

honeys compared to Manuka and multifloral honeys. *Sci Rep.* Published online 2019. doi:10.1038/s41598-019-54217-8

5. Tewari J IJ. Quantification of saccharides in multiple floral honeys using Fourier transform infrared micro attenuated total reflectance spectroscopy. Published online 2004. doi:10.1021/jf035176+

6. Andrew B Jull, Anthony Rodgers NW. Honey as a topical treatment for wounds. Published online 2008. doi:10.1002/14651858.CD005083.pub2

7. Natalia G Vallianou, Penny Gounari, Alexandros Skourtis JP and CK. Honey and its Anti-Inflammatory, Anti-Bacterial and Anti-Oxidant Properties. *Gen Med.* Published online 2014. doi:10.4172/2327-5146.1000132

8. Website N. Honey, not antibiotics, recommended for coughs. Published 2018. Accessed November 1, 2020. https://www.nhs.uk/news/heart-and-

lungs/honey-not-antibiotics-
recommended-coughs/

9. US FDA CFSAN. Voluntary Cosmetic Registration Program - Frequency of Use of Cosmetic Ingredients. Published online 2019.

10. Ganceviciene R, Liakou AI, Theodoridis A, Makrantonaki E ZC. Skin anti-aging strategies. Published online 2012. doi:10.4161/derm.22804

11. Al C et. RP-HPLC detection of water-soluble vitamins in honey. Published online 2011. doi:10.1016/j.talanta.2010.10.059

12. https://www.ncbi.nlm.nih.gov/pmc/articles/PMC6023338/.

Benefits of Honey for Weight Loss

Honey can be used as an aid to weight loss. Your diet plays an important role in your attempt to lose weight. Whatever you eat is a source of calories and may get converted into fats if not eaten in a controlled manner. Various low calorie foods are advised for people who are obese and need to lose weight. Out of those many food stuffs, there is replacement to the high calorie sugar i.e. honey. You may find many substitutes to sugar but honey is one of the natural substitutes and is not prepared out of any processing. This makes it a better choice if you are really concerned about your health. Honey has various health benefits, apart from just reducing your calorie intake.

If you feel discomfort after meals and have digestion problems, you can have honey after meals for proper digestion of food and prevention against many other stomach problems. Honey is a source of simple carbohydrates. If your food is rich in sugar or some complexes of sugars, they are carbohydrates. Being simple or complex carbohydrate depends on the stacking and binding of sugar molecules. When the sugar molecules are stacked in rows, it forms complex carbohydrates which take longer time to get digested. These types of carbohydrates are most often found in legumes and whole grains.

Talking about a source of complex carbohydrates - honey; a recent theory has enlightened a relation between weight loss and honey. A spoon full or two of honey just before sleep, either with warm water or just the honey, fuels up the liver, eases your stress hormone and assists in the fat burning process of the body. It also brings good sleep as well as helping you lose weight.

Various ways you can have honey in your diet:

With warm water: Fats, the unused resource in your body, has no use as in today's scenario. Basically, your body stores fats to be used at the time of starvation which is almost a situation that you may rarely go through. Now, the fats are nothing but a reason for you being overweight and unhealthy.

Honey has been observed to mobilise the fats and thus help in burning them for release of energy. This energy is used for various physical activities. You can have a table spoon of honey added to the same amount of warm water. It will help you in proper food digestion as well decrease your weight.

With lemon*:* Honey can also be taken along with warm water and lemon juice. Most people have this drink early in the morning believing it to help in losing belly fat.

With cinnamon*:* You can also add cinnamon powder in warm water along with honey. Mix one tablespoon of honey, one tablespoon of cinnamon powder and a cup of warm water properly and then have it on an empty stomach. Although many people have experienced weight loss with regular consumption of this mixture, it has not yet been found out as to how it brings that effect.

Honey has many other health benefits too, apart from weight loss. If you are overweight and want to lose weight, try cutting your calorie intake but make sure that you do not deprive your body of essential nutrients.

7 Ways Honey Can Make Your Life Better

Honey could *literally* save your life - yep, Manuka honey could soon be used to fight infections in hospitals, according to new research. But did you know it could also help you beat spots, lose weight and perfect your pout? Looks like Winnie the Pooh was onto something.

Read on to find out how you can reap the benefits at home. Our top tip ? Go for raw, organic varieties - heat and processing can strip honey of its health and beauty-giving enzymes and nutrients.

1. It heals (virtually) all ills.

Thanks to its antibacterial properties, honey can be used to treat minor wounds, burns and bug bites. As well as fighting infection, it forms a protective barrier and helps to reduce inflammation. It also soothes sore throats. For optimum benefits, choose Manuka honey with a UMF value of at least 10+.

2. It sorts out gnarly feet.

Honey helps to treat and prevent fungal infections. It'll also leave your trotters softer and smoother while it's at it, thanks to its moisturising properties. For a quick and easy fix, dissolve 2 tbsp. honey and a couple of drops of tea tree oil in a bowl of warm water and soak feet for 10 minutes. Feeling inspired? Whip up your own honey foot treat. Not into DIY? Try Dr Organic's Manuka Honey Foot Scrub and Foot and Heel Cream.

3. It strengthens nails.

Condition cuticles and beat brittle nails by massaging a mixture of 1 tsp honey and 1 tsp olive oil into your nails. Leave for 10 minutes before rinsing off. Up the ante ,by gently warming the mixture before applying, adding a squeeze of lemon juice to see off stains.

4. It tackles problem skin.

Yep, not only has honey been hailed a cleanser, exfoliator and moisturiser in one, it could help you beat breakouts too, thanks to its antimicrobial super powers. Gently massage a teaspoon of high quality raw honey into your face as a weekly treat, allowing it to sit on the skin for 5 minutes to reap maximum benefits. But why stop at your jawline? Stir a couple of tablespoons of honey into your bath and let those reparative and protective antioxidants get to work on the rest of you…

5. It gives you lustrous locks.

Not only will it boost shine without adding weight to dull, limp locks, but honey is said to strengthen follicles, encouraging hair growth - simply mix a teaspoon in with a squeeze of your usual shampoo. For an intensive conditioning treatment, combine 1 tablespoonful raw honey with 1 tablespoonful coconut oil and apply to ends, leaving in for up to 20 minutes before rinsing out.

6. It softens lips.

Honey's humectant properties will protect your pout from chapping (if you can refrain from licking it all off, of course). This DIY lip gloss, which combines honey with beeswax, coconut oil and your choice of essential oils, will keep you kissable all winter long…

7. It helps you lose weight (without sacrificing chocolate...)

OK, so far so good. But should you actually [gasp] eat it? It sometimes gets a bad rap on account of its sugar content, but, eaten in moderation, evidence indicates that honey could help you lose weight *and* give your health a boost. Packed with nutrients, raw honey not only lowers 'bad' cholesterol and increases 'good' cholesterol, but may help you to absorb other nutrients and even mobilise stored fats.

Swap refined sugar for honey and your blood sugar will benefit - fact. Can't face giving up chocolate? Try this genius paleo-friendly recipe for honey-sweetened homemade melt-in-your-mouth dark chocolate.

Bananas 'Better Than Sports Drinks for Athletes'

Bananas beat sports drinks as energy source for athletes, a new study has revealed.

The fruit, which is rich in potassium and nutrients, has always been a favourite for endurance runners and cyclists.

Now scientists have confirmed that as well as maintaining the same levels of energy as carbohydrate drinks, bananas also possesses healthier sugars.

The study revealed that bananas contained antioxidants not found in sugary sports drinks apart from having a greater nutritional boost.

"It shows healthier energy sources can still support an athlete's high performance," the Daily Express quoted Dr David Nieman, of Appalachian State University in North Carolina, as saying.

Double Your Energy in Just Five Days

If you're struggling to muster up enough energy to get through the day, follow these tips to boost your spirits.…

Feeling tired all the time? Can't seem to get yourself going in the morning and desperate to flop into bed at night? Follow these few simple tweaks to your daily eating habits and double your energy levels in just five days!

Eat at least two low GI meals a day

Many of the carbohydrate-based foods that we eat on a daily basis such as breads, pasta, rice, cereals, cakes and biscuits are highly processed, refined and lacking in their natural fibre therefore, once eaten, they are broken down very quickly causing our blood sugars to surge. These surges are followed by a sudden drop leaving us feeling tired, lethargic and lacking in concentration.

Research shows that swapping fast releasing, high GI (Glycemic index, measuring a food's effect on blood glucose) foods for lower GI alternatives such as wholegrain cereals, rye bread, wild or basmati rice, beans, pulses and fresh fruit and vegetables is an excellent way to significantly increase your energy. This is because they are packed with energy boosting B vitamins and they also release their sugars into your blood stream at a more constant pace throughout the day.

Iron deficiencies

Approximately 40% of women in Britain have an inadequate intake of iron and if you are one of them you may find yourself barely able to lift one foot in front of the other, feeling permanently lethargic, grumpy, lacking in motivation and concentration. Eating more iron-rich foods is one of the most significant energy-boosting moves you can make. This is because iron is essential in transporting oxygen via red blood cells to wherever it's needed in the body and without oxygen it's impossible to create energy.

Good sources of iron include liver, lean red meats, oysters, clams, tuna, salmon, beans, lentils and green leafy vegetables.

To maximise your ability to absorb iron from foods it's a good idea to eat foods rich in Vitamin C and Iron within the same meal such as a glass of fresh orange juice with your iron fortified breakfast cereal or adding tinned tomatoes to beef mince when making chilli or bolognaise.

Cut back on fatty foods

Gram for gram, fat contains more than double the amount of energy provided by protein or carbohydrates. Therefore, it may seem logical that a high fat diet should actual increase our energy levels. However, research shows the reverse to be true. This is because a diet rich in fat inhibits the body's natural ability to burn oxygen and therefore results in us feeling sluggish and lethargic.

Graze don't gorge

A skimpy breakfast, a hurried lunch, and a huge evening feast are about the least energy-efficient eating schedule imaginable. *Instead, eat a good sized breakfast, a moderate lunch and supper and add in a mid-morning and mid-afternoon snack such as a piece of fruit or a handful of mixed nuts and seeds*. Eating little and often is a great way to prevent tiredness as it provides your body with energy as and when it needs it throughout the day.

Get active

Getting active may be the last thing you feel like doing when you're tired and rung out but the phrase 'energy makes energy' really is true. This is because, the fitter you are the more efficient your heart and lungs will be at getting oxygen into and around your body – and the more oxygen you can take in and utilise the more energy you can create so do some form of cardiovascular exercise whether it's cycling, dancing, swimming, running or walking for at least 30 minutes five times a week.

Drink at least two litres of water every day

Strong tea, coffee and alcohol will not only impair your body's ability to sleep and absorb essential energy producing vitamins and minerals but they may leave you dehydrated too. Dehydration results in reduced blood volume which ultimately means your ability to transport all the essential ingredients for energy such as blood sugars (glucose), iron, and oxygen around your body is greatly reduced leaving you feeling tired, heavy and apathetic.

Five-A-Day: Fruit and Veg Portions Explained

Eating five portions of fruit and veg a day increases life expectancy and keeps you healthier for longer - but are you getting your portions right?

If you valiantly try to scoff down five portions of fruit and vegetables a day as recommended by government health officials, take heart - you're adding years to your life.

New research has found that eating your five a day increases life expectancy by around three years and even managing just three a day can give you an 18 month advantage over those who didn't eat fruit and veg every day. Fruit and veg can add years to your life.

The researchers at the Karolinska Institute in Stockholm, Sweden said their findings backed up the World Health Organisation's recommendations that we should all eat at least 400g of fruit and veg a day.

But, as we all know, it's not always that easy. Five portions is actually quite a lot and many nutritionists actually suggest we aim for more like eight portions, with five of those being vegetables. It can also be hard to tell what counts as a full portion and which vegetables count?

Five a day: The facts

You can work out what a single portion of fruit is by eye. You need about a handful of small fruits to add up to one serving. For example, two kiwis, two satsumas or two plums and for even smaller fruits such as berries and cherries, a portion is more like seven or eight.

For larger fruits such as mangoes and melons, half of the full fruit counts as a portion. A portion of veg is around the size of your palm for uncooked veggies such as raw broccoli florets or carrots. Once cooked, a measure of three heaped tablespoons counts as a portion, peas for example.

Vegetables that don't count include potatoes, which are classed as starchy carbs. Yams and plantains also fit into the category. Onions and mushrooms do count, though. Eat your greens - and stay healthier for longer.

Tinned, dried, frozen or fresh?

Fruit and veg are available in various states. Frozen veggies are thought to be even better than fresh as they retain many of their nutrients that fresh food loses in its journey from field to plate.

Tinned aren't as good as fresh or frozen but last longer and are cheaper which makes their nutrients good value for money. Both tinned and frozen should be eaten in the same portion sizes as fresh.

Take care with dried fruits as they shrink but still contain the same amount of sugar. One portion of dried fruit would be about one tablespoon of small fruits such as raisins or a handful of bigger fruits, such as banana slices.

Beans and pulses

Beans, lentils and pulses all come under the five a day umbrella. Three heaped tablespoons of cooked beans counts as a portion. However, no matter how many varieties of bean or lentil you eat, they will only count as one every day.

Juice and smoothies

Fruit juices contain antioxidants and vitamins but also high levels of natural sugar.

The craze for turning our fruit and veg to liquid seems to be here to stay but nutritionists recommend you don't drink more than one glass of fruit juice or a smoothie a day.

They're great if you're short on time and will count as one of your five-a-day but they aren't as good for you as eating the fruits whole, as they the juicing process breaks down much of the fibre.

Fruits cut depression risk by a fifth

Eating plenty of fruit reduces the risk of depression in later life, according to new research. The 20-year study involving more than 13,000 participants showed that higher consumption of fruits - including oranges, tangerines and bananas - was associated with lower chances of depressive symptoms in old age.

Eating at least three servings of fruit a day in middle age reduced the likelihood of ageing-related depression by at least 21% compared to eating one or less daily portion, say scientists. Doctors worldwide have noted an increased prevalence of depressive symptoms among older adults - including depressed feelings, lack of pleasure and delayed cognitive processing - often accompanied by loss of appetite, insomnia, poor concentration, and increased fatigue as people live longer.

They say it is related to underlying neurodegenerative changes in the brain associated with ageing. The drive to keep older adults in good health has triggered extensive research into approaches that could prevent later-life depression.

Accumulating evidence has revealed the plausible role of dietary factors in protecting against depression in ageing. The new research, conducted by the Yong Loo Lin School of Medicine at the National University of Singapore, involved 13,738 participants from the Singapore Chinese Health Study, tracked participants through their mid-life to later life spanning 20 yrs.

The research team found that participants who consumed higher quantities of fruit earlier in life exhibited a reduced likelihood of experiencing depressive symptoms later in life. The researchers studied a total of 14 fruits most commonly eaten in Singapore and found that the consumption of most fruits - including oranges, tangerines, bananas, papayas, watermelons, apple and honey melon - was associated with reduced likelihood of depression.

They say the high levels of antioxidants and anti-inflammatory micronutrients in fruits - such as vitamin C, carotenoids and flavonoids - which have been shown to reduce oxidative stress and inhibit inflammatory processes in the body may affect the development of depression.

But consumption of vegetables was found to have no association with the likelihood of depressive symptoms. The researchers say their findings, published in the Journal of Nutrition, Health and Ageing, provide "valuable insights" into the potential benefits of eating sufficient fruit in mitigating depressive symptoms later in life.

Principal investigator Professor Koh Woon Puay, of NUS Medicine, said: "Our study underscores the importance of fruit consumption as a preventive measure against ageing-related depression. In our study population, participants who had at least three servings of fruits a day, compared to those with less than one serving a day, were able to reduce the likelihood of ageing-related depression significantly by at least 21%."

"This can be achieved by eating one to two servings of fruits after every meal. We did not see any difference in our results between fruits with high and low glycaemic index. Hence, for those with diabetes, they can choose fruits with low glycaemic index that will not raise blood sugars as much as those with high index."

At the initial stage of the study from 1993 to 1998, when participants were an average age of 51, they were asked to answer a questionnaire on how often they consumed a standard serving size of each food item daily, for 14 fruits and 25 vegetables. In 2014 to 2016, when participants were an average age of 73, depressive symptoms were examined using a standard test and 3,180 (23.1%) participants who reported having five or more symptoms were considered to have depression.

After adjusting for factors including medical history, smoking status, level of physical activity and sleep duration, the researchers found that higher consumption of fruits, but not vegetables, was associated with lower odds of depressive symptoms. Prof Koh said: "Our study aimed to examine the relationship of mid-life consumption of fruits and vegetables with the risk of depressive symptoms in late life."

"Although other studies have also examined the associations of fruits and vegetables with risk of depression, there are inconsistencies in the results."

She added: "These findings suggest that promoting fruit consumption for individuals in mid adulthood, typically defined as ages 40 to 65, could yield long-term benefits for their mental well-being at late adulthood beyond 65."

The research team is now looking into the association of other modifiable behaviours - such as sleep duration, smoking and other dietary factors - with the mental health of older adults.

Five Surprisingly Healthy Foods

Everyday foods with surprising health benefits

Some foods' health benefits are shouted from the roof tops and make us feel smug every time we munch on them.

Everyday foods such as green tea, chillies and chocolate have well-documented health benefits but there are some lesser-known healthy foods that haven't had the praise they deserve.

Here are five unlikely foods and drinks that can benefit health, when eaten as part of a balanced diet. Did you know about them?

Popcorn

This fluffy snack has a lot more to offer than just something to nibble on at the cinema.

We've known for a while that popcorn is low in calories, but scientists have found some other benefits to eating it. Joe Vinson and his team from the University of Scranton in Pennsylvania found that popcorn contains concentrated levels of antioxidants, due to its low water content.

However, popcorn toppings can contain hidden calories. Researchers stated that air-popped popcorn had the lowest calories, while microwave popcorn contained twice as many, and as much as 43 per cent fat. To get the most out of popcorn, go for the air-popped varieties without lots of salt, sugar or toffee glaze.

Black Tea

Up until recently, green tea seemed to get all the 'health' headlines. But drinking black tea can also benefit your health too.

In one Iranian study, researchers found that participants who drank more than three cups of black tea daily had a 70 per cent lower risk of coronary artery disease. And a study carried out in the Netherlands found that just two servings of black tea per day improved brain function and focused attention. Better get the kettle on, then.

Coffee

It's refreshing, it wakes you up and too much of it might give you the shakes. But a 2012 study found that coffee could also help protect against certain forms of cancer.

The 26-year study found those who drank four or more cups of coffee each day were 50 per cent less likely to die from mouth or throat cancers. The researchers concluded by saying, 'there may be beneficial effects to coffee, particularly caffeinated coffee and its daily enjoyment.'

But that's not all. A joint study by the University of South Florida and the University of Miami found a link between drinking coffee and the onset of Alzheimer's.

'We are not saying that moderate coffee consumption will completely protect people from Alzheimer's disease,' lead author of the study

Chuanhai Cao said, 'however we firmly believe that moderate coffee consumption can appreciably reduce your risk of Alzheimer's or delay its onset.'

Eggs

For a long time, eggs tended to get a bad rep because of worries over cholesterol. But health experts now agree that it's saturated fat intake and not dietary cholesterol which we should watch for a healthy heart.

Eggs contain many vitamins and minerals that are essential to health, including folate, calcium, iron and selenium. They also help you feel fuller for longer and contain choline - important for memory and brain function, as well as helping to maintain a healthy liver.

Cheese

In 2011, researchers at Copenhagen University studied the effects of a cheese-rich diet on levels of LDL (bad) cholesterol. They found that when people ate a set (but regular) amount of cheese for six weeks, their LDL cholesterol levels did not increase, and actually lowered when they switched from a butter-rich diet to eating cheese.

Researchers think that because cheese contains high levels of protein and calcium, our bodies find it easier to break down the cholesterol.

But, unfortunately, this isn't an excuse to suddenly eat lots of cheese - participants ate cheese instead of other fats in their diet, and not to excess. It's worth remembering that it is still a fatty food, and should be eaten in moderation.

Food Advice

There's not a day that goes by when someone doesn't come to us asking for diet advice confused as to why they're NOT losing weight even though they don't eat "a lot"...and even if they're eating "healthy". The truth is that while "quantity" does matter, it's possible to still overconsume calories if choosing the wrong foods.

Some foods, even though they're considered very healthy, they carry loads of calories in a very small amount of food. We call these calorically dense foods and if your diet is comprised of a bunch of them, you can easily gain weight even without eating "a lot" of food.

Here are some "healthy" examples of calorically dense foods:

1. Granola - granola, especially the varieties mixed with nuts can pack as many as 500 calories per cup!

2. Pasta - a moderate 1 and 1/2 cups of most pastas yield more than 60 grams of carbs and almost 350 calories.

3. Avocado - avocado is awesome and a great source of monounsaturated fat, but one single avocado is over 300 calories and 30 grams of fat.

4. Nuts and Nut Butters - nuts are super healthy, but one of the most calorically dense foods around. A few ounces could mean more than 400 calories.

5. Fruit Juice and Smoothies - all fruit juices are loaded with sugar and so are most "smoothie" shop smoothies (make your own with whole fruit).

6. Dried Fruit - dried fruits remove the water content which dramatically decreases volume, what's left is high in sugar and very calorically dense.

7. "Whole Wheat" Breads - even the 100% whole wheat variety can pack a mean calorie punch if you're eating a lot of grains as part of your diet.

8. Whole Grain Bagels - a large "deli" bagel is loaded with carbs and calories, many times over 400 calories in a single bagel.

While some of the foods above are only "thought" to be healthy (fruit juice, whole grain bagels, etc.), stuff like nuts, nut butters, and avocado are foods that I'd recommend in just about everyone's diet and they are indeed great choices.

That said, these calorically dense foods require that you monitor your intake of them closely. A few ounces of nuts, a couple tablespoons of nut butter, and an avocado is NOT a lot of food, but if you ate all of these every day, you'd be getting close to 1000 calories just right there.

Japanese doctor who lived to 105; his Spartan diet, views on retirement, and other rare longevity tips

Dr Shigeaki Hinohara had an extraordinary life for many reasons. For starters, the Japanese physician and longevity expert lived until the age of 105.

When he died, in 2017, Hinohara was chairman emeritus of St. Luke's International University and honorary president of St. Luke's International Hospital, both in Tokyo.

Perhaps best known for his book, "Living Long, Living Good," Hinohara offered advice that helped make Japan the world leader in longevity. Some were fairly intuitive points, while others were less obvious:

1. Don't retire. But if you must, do so a lot later than age 65.

The average retirement age, at least in the U.S., has always hovered at around 65. And, in recent years, many have embraced the FIRE movement (Financial Independence, Retire Early).

But Hinohara viewed things differently. "There is no need to ever retire, but if one must, it should be a lot later than 65," he said in a 2009 interview with The Japan Times. "The current retirement age was set at 65 half a century ago, when the average life expectancy in Japan was 68 years and only 125 Japanese were over 100 years old."

Today, he explained, people are living a lot longer. The life expectancy for U.S. in 2020, for example, is 78.93 years, a 0.08% increase from 2019. Therefore, we should be retiring much later in life, too.

Hinohara certainly practiced what he preached: Until a few months before his death, he continued to treat patients, kept an appointment book with space for five more years, and worked up to 18 hours a day.

2. Take the stairs (and keep your weight in check).

Hinohara emphasized the importance of regular exercise. "I take two stairs at a time, to get my muscles moving," he said.

Additionally, Hinohara carried his own packages and luggage, and gave 150 lectures a year, usually speaking for 60 to 90 minutes — all done standing, he said, "to stay strong."

He also pointed out that people who live an extremely long life have a commonality: They aren't overweight. Indeed, obesity is widely considered one of the most significant risk factors for increased morbidity and mortality.

Hinohara's diet was Spartan: "For breakfast, I drink coffee, a glass of milk and some orange juice with a tablespoon of olive oil in it." (Studies have found that olive oil offers numerous health benefits, such as keeping your arteries clean and lowering heart disease risk.)

"Lunch is milk and a few cookies, or nothing when I am too busy to eat," he continued. "I never get hungry because I focus on my work. Dinner is veggies, a bit of fish and rice, and, twice a week, 100 grams of lean meat."

3. Find a purpose that keeps you busy.

According to Hinohara, not having a full schedule is a sure-fire way to age faster and die sooner. However, it's important to stay busy not just for the *sake* of staying busy, but to be active in activities that help serve a purpose. (The logic is that one can be busy, yet still feel empty and idle on the inside.)

Hinohara found his purpose early on, after his mother's life was saved by the family's doctor.

Janit Kawaguchi, a journalist who considered Hinohara a mentor, said, "He believed that life is all about contribution, so he had this incredible drive to help people, to wake up early in the morning and do something wonderful for other people. This is what was driving him and what kept him living."

"It's wonderful to live long," Hinohara said in the interview. "Until one is 60 years old, it is easy to work for one's family and to achieve one's goals. But in our later years, we should strive to contribute to society. Since the age of 65, I have worked as a volunteer. I still put in 18 hours seven days a week and love every minute of it."

4. Rules are stressful; try to relax them.

While he clearly promoted exercise and nutrition as pathways to a longer and healthier life, Hinohara simultaneously maintained that we need not be obsessed with restricting our behaviours.

"We all remember how, as children, when we were having fun, we would forget to eat or sleep," he often said. "I believe we can keep that attitude as adults — it is best not to tire the body with too many rules."

Richard Overton, one of America's oldest-surviving World War II veterans, would have most likely agreed. Right up until his death at age 112, the supercentenarian smoked cigars, drank whisky and ate fried food and ice cream on a daily basis.

Hinohara might not have approved of Overton's diet, but, to be fair, Overton did credit his longevity to maintaining a "stress-free life and keeping busy."

5. Remember that doctors can't cure everything.

Hinohara cautioned against always taking the doctor's advice. When a test or surgery is recommended, he advised, "Ask whether the doctor would suggest that his or her spouse or children go through such a procedure."

Hinohara insisted that science alone can't help people. It "lumps us all together, but illness is individual. Each person is unique, and diseases are connected to their hearts," he said. "To know the illness and help people, we need liberal and visual arts, not just medical ones."

In fact, Hinohara made sure that St. Luke's catered to the basic need of patients: "To have fun." The hospital provided music, animal therapy and art classes.

"Pain is mysterious, and having fun is the best way to forget it," he said. "If a child has a toothache, and you start playing a game together, he or she immediately forgets the pain."

6. Find inspiration, joy and peace in art.

According to The New York Times, toward the end of his life, Hinohara was unable to eat, but refused a feeding tube. He was discharged and died months later at home.

Instead of trying to fight death, Hinohara found peace in where he was through art. In fact, he credited his contentment and outlook toward life to a poem by Robert Browning, called "Abt Vogler", especially these lines:

There shall never be one lost good! What was, shall live as before; The evil is null, is nought, is silence implying sound; What was good shall be good, with, for evil, so much good more; On the earth the broken arcs; in the heaven a perfect round.

"My father used to read it to me," Hinohara recalled. "It encourages us to make big art, not small scribbles. It says to try to draw a circle so huge that there is no way we can finish it while we are alive. All we see is an arch; the rest is beyond our vision, but it is there in the distance."

7 Nutritious Foods That Are High in Vitamin D

(Written on "Healthline" website by Taylor Jones, RD and Medically reviewed by Imashi Fernando, MS, RDN)

We know that vitamin D affects many bodily functions, including bone health. Research also suggests that low vitamin D levels may be a risk factor for autoimmune diseases. Many people don't get enough vitamin D. It's hard to know how many people are deficient because experts are still debating about what target levels should be. Research suggests that about 24% of people in the United States are vitamin D deficient. Other areas of the world may have higher rates of deficiency. It's estimated that in Europe, about 40% of the population has vitamin D deficiency.

Our bodies produce vitamin D when exposed to sunlight. There are a few reasons why it's hard to get enough vitamin D this way. To reduce the risk of skin cancer, it's smart to cover up, wear sunscreen, and avoid being outside during peak sun hours. And depending on where you live in the world, it may just not be possible to have enough year-round sun exposure. That's why getting vitamin D from food or supplements is best.

Daily recommended dose of vitamin D

The daily value (DV) for vitamin D is 800 IU (20 mcg). The vitamin D content is listed as a percentage of the DV on the nutrition facts label on food packages. This tells you what amount of your daily vitamin D requirement the food will provide.

It's best to get vitamin D from food or supplements. Whether you need a vitamin D supplement in addition to food and sun exposure is a question to ask your doctor. They can also help you find out if you are deficient.

Natural sources

- **Salmon**

Salmon is a popular fatty fish and a great source of vitamin D. According to the United States Department of Agriculture (USDA) Food Composition Database, one 3.5-ounce (100-gram) serving of farmed Atlantic salmon contains 526 IU of vitamin D, or 66% of the DV.

Whether the salmon is wild or farmed can make a big difference in the vitamin D content. On average, wild-caught salmon has more vitamin D. The amount of vitamin D will vary depending on where the salmon is caught and the time of year. One study showed that the vitamin D content of salmon caught in the Baltic sea ranged from 556–924 IU of vitamin D per one 3.5-ounce (100-gram) serving, providing 70–111% of the DV.

- **Herring and Sardines**

Herring is a fish eaten around the world. It is often smoked or pickled. This small fish is also a great source of vitamin D. Fresh Atlantic herring provides

214 IU per 3.5-ounce (100-gram) serving, which is 27% of the DV. If fresh fish isn't your thing, pickled herring is also a good source of vitamin D, providing 113 IU per 3.5-ounce (100-gram) serving, or 14% of the DV. Pickled herring also contains a high amount of sodium, at 870 mg per serving. It may not be a great option if you are trying to lower your salt intake of canned sardines are a good source of vitamin D as well. A 3.5-ounce (100-gram) serving provides 193 IU or 24% of the DV.

Other types of fatty fish are also good vitamin D sources. Halibut and mackerel provide 190 IU and 643 IU per 3.5-ounce (100-gram) serving, respectively.**3.**

- **Cod liver oil**

Cod liver oil is a popular supplement. If you don't like fish, taking cod liver oil is another way to get nutrients that are hard to get otherwise. It's an excellent source of vitamin D. At about 450 IU per teaspoon (4.9 mL), it clocks in at a massive 56% of the DV. It has been used for many years to treat vitamin D deficiency. It also has a history of being used as part of treating rickets, psoriasis, and tuberculosis. Cod liver oil is also very high in vitamin A, with 150% of the DV in just a single teaspoon (4.9 mL). Vitamin A can be toxic in high amounts. The safe upper limit (UL) for vitamin A is 3,000 mcg. A single teaspoon (4.9 mL) of cod liver oil contains 1,350 mcg of vitamin A. Make sure that you aren't exceeding the upper limit with cod liver oil or any other vitamin A supplements.

In addition, cod liver oil is high in omega-3 fatty acids. Omega-3s may play a role in heart health and may reduce inflammation in the body. Along with fatty fish, cod liver oil is another source of these fatty acids. If you don't eat fish, it can be hard to get enough omega-3 in your diet.

- **Canned tuna**

Many people enjoy canned tuna because of its flavour and easy storage methods. It is typically cheaper than buying fresh fish. Canned light tuna packs up to 269 IU of vitamin D in a 3.5-ounce (100-gram) serving, which is 34% of the DV. Mercury is a heavy metal found in many types of fish. Bigger types of fish contain more mercury than smaller ones. The amount of mercury in canned tuna depends on the type of tuna. Light canned tuna comes from smaller fish and is lower in mercury. White canned tuna is higher in mercury. Over time, methylmercury can build up in your body. In some cases, it can lead to serious health concerns.

The Environmental Defense Fund (EDF) recommends only a single 3.5-ounce (100-gram) serving of light tuna per week. If you're concerned about mercury consumption, talk with your doctor about the appropriate amount of tuna to eat per week for you.

- **Egg yolks**

Fish are not the only source of vitamin D. Whole eggs are another good source, as well as a wonderfully nutritious food. Most of the protein in an egg is found in the white, and the fat, vitamins, and minerals are found mostly in the yolk. The yolk from one large egg contains 37 IU of vitamin D, or 5% of the DV.

A few factors affect the vitamin D level of egg yolks. Sun exposure for the chicken, the vitamin D content of the chicken feed, and exposing liquid yolk to UV light will increase vitamin D in the egg. When given the same feed, pasture- raised chickens that roam outside in the sunlight produce eggs with levels 3–4 times higher. Additionally, eggs from chickens given vitamin D enriched feed may have up to 34,815 IU of vitamin D per 100 grams of yolk. So, if one yolk is about 17 grams, that means you'll get around 2.5 times the DV of vitamin D in a single egg. Choosing eggs either from chickens raised outside or marketed as high in vitamin D can be a great way to meet your daily requirements.

- **Mushrooms**

Other than fortified foods, mushrooms are the only sufficient non-animal source of vitamin D. Like humans, mushrooms can synthesize vitamin D when exposed to UV light. However, mushrooms produce vitamin D2, whereas animals produce vitamin D3. Though vitamin D2 helps raise blood levels of vitamin D, it may not be as effective as vitamin D3 .Some wild mushrooms are excellent sources of vitamin D2 because of their exposure to UV light. Morels are a type of mushroom that grows in the wild. One cup of these mushrooms contains 136 IU of vitamin D, which is 17% of the DV. Many commercially grown mushrooms are grown in the dark and contain very little D2. Some mushrooms are being treated with ultraviolet (UV) light to boost their vitamin D content. One cup of cremini mushrooms exposed to UV light contains 1,110 IU of vitamin D, which is 139% of the DV. Natural sources of vitamin D are limited, especially if you're vegetarian or don't like fish.

Other sources

Fortunately, some food products that don't naturally contain vitamin D are fortified with this nutrient.

- **Cow's milk**

Cow's milk is a naturally good source of many nutrients, including calcium, phosphorous, and riboflavin. In several countries, cow's milk is fortified with vitamin D. In the United States, 1 cup of fortified cow's milk contains 115 IU of vitamin D per cup (237 mL), or about 15% of the DV.

- **Soy milk**

Since vitamin D is found almost exclusively in animal products, vegetarians and vegans may find it trickier to get enough. For this reason, plant-based milk substitutes such as soy milk are often fortified with vitamin D, along with other nutrients usually found in cow's milk. The amount can vary depending on the brand. One cup (237 mL) contains around 100–119 IU of vitamin D, or 13–15% of the DV.

- **Orange juice**

Around 65% of people worldwide are lactose intolerant, and around 2% have a milk allergy. For this reason, some companies fortify orange juice with vitamin D and other nutrients, such as calcium. One cup (237 mL) of fortified orange juice with breakfast can start your day off with up to 100 IU of vitamin D, or 12% of the DV. However, orange juice isn't a great option for everyone. For people prone to acid reflux, it can worsen symptoms. If you live with diabetes, you may notice that juice causes a spike in your blood sugar level. That said, it's a great option if you're trying to treat a low blood sugar level.

- **Cereal and oatmeal**

Cereals are another food that may be fortified with vitamin D. One cup of fortified wheat bran flakes contains 145 IU of vitamin D, equal to 18% of the DV. One cup of fortified crisp rice cereal has 85 IU of vitamin D, or 11% of the DV. Remember that not all cereals will contain vitamin D. It's smart to check the nutrition label to find out how much vitamin D is in the product. Though fortified cereals and oatmeal provide less vitamin D than many natural sources, they can still be a good way to boost your intake.

Vitamin D and Calcium

Vitamin D is necessary for calcium absorption in your body. This plays a key role in maintaining bone strength and skeletal integrity. Getting enough of both vitamin D and calcium is crucial to maintaining bone health and protecting against disorders like osteoporosis, a condition that is characterized by weak, brittle bones. While the daily value (DV) of vitamin D is 800 IU per day, the recommended dietary allowance (RDA) differs slightly depending on your age. Children and adults ages 1–70 need approximately 600 IU of vitamin D per day. This can come from a combination of food sources and sunlight. Adults over 70 should aim for at least 800 IU (20 mcg) of vitamin D per day. The RDA for calcium also varies by age. Children ages 4–8 need about 1,000 mg of calcium daily. Children ages 9–18 need approximately 1,300 mg daily. Adults ages 19–50 need about 1,000 mg daily. Over the age of 50, most people need 1,200 mg per day.

Conclusion

Although our bodies can make vitamin D from UV light from the sun, that's not necessarily the best way to meet your needs. The Centres for Disease Control (CDC) recommend several steps to limit UV exposure to reduce the risk of skin cancer. These include spending more time in the shade, wearing sunscreen, and covering up when you are in the sun. Because of this, food sources of vitamin D or vitamin D supplements are typically the best way to consistently and safely meet your vitamin D needs.

Getting enough vitamin D from your diet alone may be difficult, but not impossible. The foods listed in this article are some of the top sources of vitamin D available. Eating plenty of these foods rich in vitamin D is a great way to make sure you get enough of this important nutrient.

Healthy Food

A varied, balanced diet is the cornerstone of healthy living for everyone, yet healthy eating can sometimes mean different things depending on your gender. While there are some foods we should all be eating more of, men and women also have their own set of dietary requirements as well as their own unique health concerns. Here are ten foods all men should eat.

1) Blueberries

Blueberries are another fruit that have been linked to a reduced risk of prostate cancer, thanks to their high levels of proanthocyanidins. However, blueberries' positive benefits for men don't stop there, as studies have also suggested that blueberries may be effective in reducing risk of heart disease, Type 2

Diabetes and age-related memory loss; a condition more prevalent in men than women.

2) Whole grains

Whole grains are great for our health thanks to their high levels of vitamins, minerals and fibre. Most whole grains, including brown rice and oats, are particularly rich in B vitamins, which are good for general wellbeing and can also help alleviate depression. Individual B vitamins can also benefit male health in various ways. Studies have suggested that folate (vitamin B9) can keep sperm healthy, while biotin (B7) may help hair loss. Silica, also present in whole grains, could also help with healthy hair growth.

3) Brazil nuts

Snacking on nuts is great for heart health and good skin. However, Brazil nuts are particularly beneficial for men as they are packed with selenium; a powerful antioxidant which studies have suggested can boost sperm health and motility. Furthermore, selenium is also great for lowering "bad" cholesterol levels, preventing blood clots and lifting your mood.

4) Broccoli

Broccoli - along with other cruciferous vegetables like cabbage and sprouts – contain a strong cancer-fighting chemical, sulphoraphane, which research has suggested may reduce men's risk of developing bladder cancer (a cancer more commonly affecting women than men), prostate cancer and colorectal cancer.

5) Oysters

Oysters are the highest natural source of zinc; an essential requirement for men's fertility and sexual health. Zinc not only helps to maintain healthy testosterone levels in men, but it is essential for healthy sperm production. On top of this, zinc deficiency may be responsible for hair loss in men, so an increased intake may benefit men's appearance as well as health.

6) Tomatoes

Tomatoes are possibly one of the best "super foods" around, and the popular fruit has particular benefits for men. Studies have suggested that the lycopene found in tomatoes may reduce risk of colorectal cancer, lower cholesterol and reduce the risk of heart disease; the leading cause of death in men. Research has also shown that men who frequently eat foods rich in lycopene may drastically reduce their risk of developing prostate cancer.

7) Eggs

For men suffering from hair loss, eggs may also provide the perfect solution. Eggs are an excellent source of protein, which is essential for hair growth, as well as being rich in biotin (vitamin B7). Egg yolks are also a good source of iron, which some studies have suggested can alleviate hair loss, which can be caused by anaemia.

8) Pomegranate juice

Pomegranates are packed with antioxidants, vitamins and minerals, and research has suggested that drinking the juice of this "super food" can help lower cholesterol - which can be high in many men as young as their 20s - and prevent hypertension. A study has also found that drinking just one 8oz glass of pomegranate juice a day could dramatically slow down the progress of prostate cancer.

9) Garlic

Garlic is well known for boosting heart health, and a study on the effects of garlic consumption on males has shown that regularly eating garlic could help lower men's cholesterol levels. Furthermore, research findings published in the Journal of the National Cancer Institute have suggested that regularly eating garlic and onions could help lower men's risk of developing prostate cancer.

10) Salmon

Salmon is not only a great source of protein, but it is an excellent source of omega-3 fatty acids, which can help address many of men's most common health complaints. Omega-3 fatty acids have been linked to lowered levels of "bad" cholesterol and can also reduce risk of many illnesses, including heart disease, colorectal cancer, prostate cancer and depression.

Coffee Reduces Alzheimer's Risk in Elderly

Drinking coffee every day can do more than just keeping you alert - especially if you're an older adult.

A recent study monitoring the memory and thinking processes of people older than 65, found that all those with higher blood caffeine levels avoided the onset of Alzheimer's disease in the two-to-four years of study follow-up.

And coffee appeared to be the major or only source of caffeine for these individuals.

Researchers from the University of South Florida and the University of Miami said the case control study provides the first direct evidence that caffeine/coffee intake is associated with a reduced risk of dementia or delayed onset. The collaborative study involved 124 people, ages 65 to 88, in Tampa and Miami.

"These intriguing results suggest that older adults with mild memory impairment who drink moderate levels of coffee -- about 3 cups a day -- will not convert to Alzheimer's disease -- or at least will experience a substantial delay before converting to Alzheimer's," said study lead author Dr Chuanhai Cao, a neuroscientist at the USF College of Pharmacy and the USF Health Byrd Alzheimer's Institute.

Dr Cao stated "The results from this study, along with our earlier studies in Alzheimer's mice, are very consistent in indicating that moderate daily caffeine/coffee intake throughout adulthood should appreciably protect against Alzheimer's disease later in life".

The study showed this protection probably occurs even in older people with early signs of the disease, called *mild cognitive impairment (MCI)*.

Patients with MCI already experience some short-term memory loss and initial Alzheimer's pathology in their brains. Each year, about 15 per cent of MCI patients progress to full-blown Alzheimer's disease.

The researchers focused on study participants with MCI, because many were destined to develop Alzheimer's within a few years.

Blood caffeine levels at the study's onset were substantially lower (51 per cent less) in participants diagnosed with MCI who progressed to dementia during the two-to-four year follow-up than in those whose mild cognitive impairment remained stable over the same period.

No one with MCI who later developed Alzheimer's had initial blood caffeine levels above a critical level of 1200 ng/ml - equivalent to drinking several cups of coffee a few hours before the blood sample was drawn. In contrast, many with stable MCI had blood caffeine levels higher than this critical level.

"We found that 100 per cent of the MCI patients with plasma caffeine levels above the critical level experienced no conversion to Alzheimer's disease during the two-to-four year follow-up period," said study co-author Dr Gary Arendash.

The researchers believe higher blood caffeine levels indicate habitually higher caffeine intake, most probably through coffee. Caffeinated coffee appeared to be the main, if not exclusive, source of caffeine in the memory-protected MCI patients, because they had the same profile of blood immune markers as Alzheimer's mice given caffeinated coffee.

Dr Cao cautioned "We are not saying that moderate coffee consumption will completely protect people from Alzheimer's disease. However, we firmly believe that moderate coffee consumption can appreciably reduce your risk of Alzheimer's or delay its onset."

Their findings will appear in the online version of an article to be published June 5 in the Journal of Alzheimer's Disease, published by IOS Press.

Potatoes Are a Good Source of Potassium

There are many ways to eat potatoes, we eat them mashed or fried, and despite our love for them, we always hear negative information about them. For example, that they contain a high percentage of carbohydrates and perhaps this is what makes many people avoid them in their diet for fear of gaining weight or high blood sugar.

Nutritionist Sarah Garone mentioned in her report published by the American magazine *"Eat This"*, that it has been advised by many, to stay away from potatoes because they are unhealthy, while in fact they are rich in many nutrients which are beneficial to the body, especially potassium. Potassium regulates blood pressure, and thus reduces the risk of cardiovascular disease. It was found that the higher the proportion of sodium to potassium in the body, the greater the risk of cardiovascular disease. She explained that potassium helps reduce the bad effect of sodium on blood pressure. According to many centres for Disease Control and Prevention, increasing potassium consumption can lower the risk of heart disease by lowering blood pressure.

The author pointed out that Americans suffer from a chronic deficiency of potassium. Since 2012, less than 2% of adults in the United States consumed the recommended daily amount of potassium, which is 4.7 grams. Potassium can improve your general health, not just your heart and getting enough potassium improves nerve and muscle function and prevents kidney stones.

The percentage of potassium in potatoes varies according to its size and the soil in which it was grown. According to the US Department of Agriculture, one baked medium sized potato contains 952 milligrams of potassium, which is 20% of the recommended daily allowance for adults.

To sum up, potatoes are one of the foods that contain high potassium content, and like all starchy vegetables it is recommended to eat them without adding salt, in order to get the most benefit.

It is Not the Saturated Fat Which Clogs the Arteries: Coronary Heart Disease Is a Chronic Inflammatory Condition

A survey published in the British Journal of Sports Medicine (2017), conducted by Aseem Malhotra, Rita F Redberg and Pascal Meier, from the Academy of Medical Royal Colleges, University of California (San Francisco) and University College (London).

They believe that coronary artery disease pathogenesis and treatment urgently requires a paradigm shift. Despite popular belief among doctors and the public, the conceptual model of dietary saturated fat clogging a pipe is just plain wrong. A landmark systematic review and meta-analysis of observational studies showed no association between saturated fat consumption and (1) all-cause mortality, (2) coronary heart disease (CHD), (3) CHD mortality, (4) ischaemic stroke or

(5) type 2 diabetes in healthy adults.[1] Similarly in the secondary prevention of CHD there is no benefit from reduced fat, including saturated fat, on myocardial infarction, cardiovascular or all-cause mortality.[2] It is instructive to note that in an angiographic study of postmenopausal women with CHD, greater intake of saturated fat was associated with less progression of atherosclerosis whereas carbohydrate and polyunsaturated fat intake were associated with greater progression.[3]

Preventing the development of atherosclerosis is important but it is atherothrombosis that is the real killer:

The inflammatory processes that contribute to cholesterol deposition within the artery wall and subsequent plaque formation (atherosclerosis), more closely resembles a 'pimple' (figure 1). Most cardiac events occur at sites with less than 70% coronary artery obstruction and these do not generate ischaemia on stress testing.[4] When plaques rupture (analogous to a pimple bursting), coronary thrombosis and myocardial infarction can occur within minutes. The limitation of the current plumbing approach ('unclogging a pipe') to the management of coronary disease is revealed by a series of *randomised controlled trials (RCTs)* which prove that stenting significantly obstructive stable lesions fail to prevent myocardial infarction or to reduce mortality.[5]

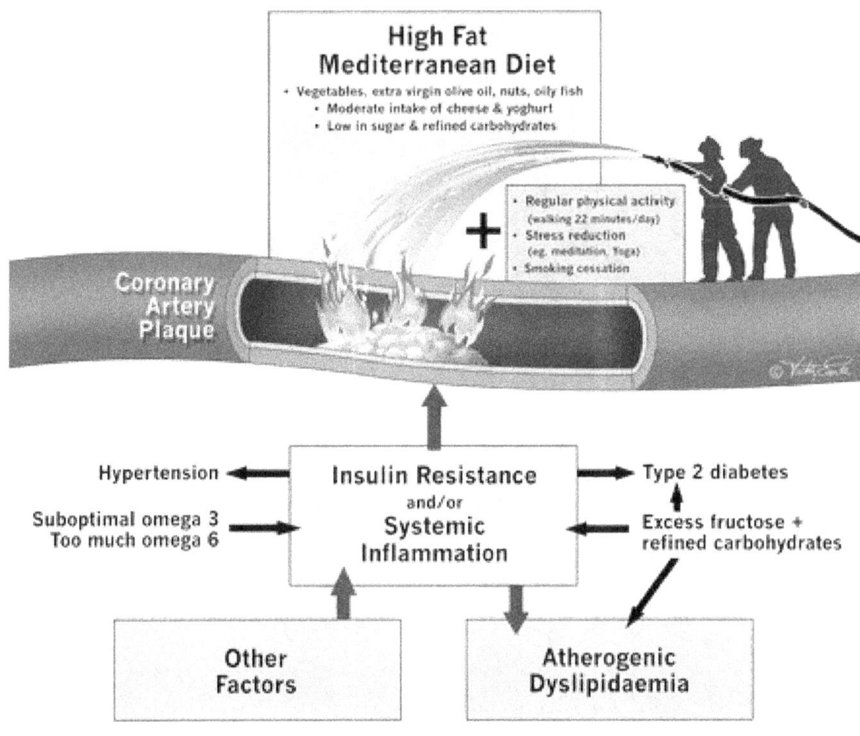

Figure 1

Lifestyle interventions for the prevention and treatment of coronary disease

Dietary Randomised Controlled Trials (TRC) with outcome benefit in primary and secondary prevention:

In comparison with advice to follow a 'low fat' diet (37% fat), an energy-unrestricted Mediterranean diet (41% fat) supplemented with at least four tablespoons of extra virgin olive oil or a handful of nuts achieved a significant 30% (Number Needed to Treat (NNT) = 61) reduction in cardiovascular events in over 7500 high-risk patients. Furthermore, the Lyon Heart study showed that adopting a Mediterranean diet in secondary prevention improved hard outcomes for both recurrent myocardial infarction (NNT=18) and all-cause mortality (NNT=30), despite there being no significant difference in plasma low-density lipoprotein (LDL) cholesterol between the two groups. It is the alpha linoleic acid, polyphenols and omega-3 fatty acids present in nuts, extra virgin olive oil, vegetables and oily fish that rapidly attenuate inflammation and coronary thrombosis.[6] Both control diets in these studies were relatively healthy, which make it highly likely that even larger benefits would be observed if the Mediterranean diets discussed above were compared with a typical western diet.

LDL cholesterol risk has been exaggerated:

Decades of emphasis on the primacy of lowering plasma cholesterol, as if this was an end in itself and driving a market of 'proven to lower cholesterol' and 'low-fat' foods and medications, has been misguided. Selective reporting may partly explain this misconception. Reanalysis of unpublished data from the Sydney Diet Heart Study and the Minnesota coronary experiment reveal replacing saturated fat with linoleic acid containing vegetable oils increased mortality risk despite significant reductions in LDL and total cholesterol (TC).[7]

A high TC to high-density lipoprotein (HDL) ratio is the best predictor of cardiovascular risk (hence this calculation, not LDL, is used in recognised cardiovascular risk calculators such as that from Framingham). A high TC to HDL ratio is also a surrogate marker for insulin resistance (i.e. chronically elevated serum insulin at the root of heart disease, type 2 diabetes and obesity). And in those over 60 years, a recent systematic review concluded that LDL cholesterol is not associated with cardiovascular disease and is inversely associated with all-cause mortality.[8] A high TC to HDL ratio drops rapidly with dietary changes such as replacing refined carbohydrates with healthy high fat foods.

A simple way to combat insulin resistance (chronically high levels of serum insulin) and inflammation:

Compared with physically inactive individuals, those who walk briskly at or above 150 min/week can increase life expectancy by 3.4–4.5 years independent of body weight.[9] Regular brisk walking may also be more effective than running in preventing coronary disease. And just 30 min of moderate activity a day more than three times/week significantly improves insulin sensitivity and helps reverse insulin resistance (i.e., lowers the chronically elevated levels of insulin that are associated with obesity) within months in sedentary middle-aged adults. This occurs, independent of weight loss and suggests even a little activity goes a long way.

Another risk factor for CHD (Chronic Heart Disease) is environmental stress. Childhood trauma can lead to an average decrease in life expectancy of 20 years. Chronic stress increases glucocorticoid receptor resistance, which results in failure to down regulate the inflammatory response. Combining a complete lifestyle approach of a healthful diet, regular movement and stress reduction will improve quality of life; reduce cardiovascular and all-cause mortality.[10] It is time to shift the public health message in the prevention and treatment of coronary artery disease away from measuring serum lipids and reducing dietary saturated fat. Coronary artery disease is a chronic inflammatory disease, and it can be reduced effectively by walking 22 min a day and eating real food. There is no business model or market to help spread this simple yet powerful intervention.

References

1. *Intake of saturated and trans unsaturated fatty acids and risk of all-cause mortality, cardiovascular disease, and type 2 diabetes: systematic review and meta-analysis of observational studies. BMJ 2015;351:h3978.doi:10.1136/bmj.h3978*

2. *Dietary fatty acids in the secondary prevention of coronary heart disease: a systematic review, meta-analysis and meta-regression. BMJ Open 2014;4:e004487.doi:10.1136/bmjopen-2013-004487*

3. *Dietary fats, carbohydrate, and progression of coronary atherosclerosis in*

postmenopausal women. *Am J Clin Nutr* 2004;80:1175–84.

4. *Coronary artery disease as clogged pipes: a misconceptual model. Circ Cardiovasc Qual Outcomes 2013;6:129–32.doi:10.1161/CIRCOUTCOMES.112.967778*

5. *The whole truth about coronary stents: the elephant in the room. JAMA Intern Med 2014;174:1367–8.doi:10.1001/jamainternmed.2013.9190*

6. *Review: nutriceuticals as antithrombotic agents. Cardiovasc Ther 2010;28:227–35.doi:10.1111/j.1755-5922.2010.00161.x*

7. *Re-evaluation of the traditional diet-heart hypothesis: analysis of recovered data from Minnesota coronary experiment (1968-73). BMJ 2016;353:i1246.doi:10.1136/bmj.i1246*

8. *Lack of an association or an inverse association between low-density-lipoprotein cholesterol and mortality in the elderly: a systematic review. BMJ Open 2016;6:e010401.doi:10.1136/bmjopen-2015-010401*

9. *Leisure time physical activity of moderate to vigorous intensity and mortality: a large pooled cohort analysis. PLoS Med*

2012;9:e1001335.doi:10.1371/journal.pmed.1001335

10. *Too toxic to ignore. Nature 2012;490:169–71.*

9 798629 059769